W9-BRT-982

HYPOGLYCEMIA

A NUTRITIONAL APPROACH

by
Louise Tenney, M.H.

Published by
Woodland Books

Printed in U.S.A.

HYPOGLYCEMIA

"The American Sugar Syndrome"

Hypoglycemia means low blood sugar. Hypo means "low" and glycemia means "sugar". It is associated with "highs" and "lows". Mood swings switch drastically from feeling happy and energetic to being anxious, irritable, tearful and depressed with mental confusion and manifestation of phobias. Hypoglycemia is also referred to as hypoadrenocorticism (low functioning adrenal glands), "hyperinsulinism" (excessive insulin) and "neuroglycopenia" (lack of sugar within the brain cells).

The most common form of hypoglycemia (functional) was first recognized in 1924 by Dr. Seale Harris. He discovered this condition when he was treating patients who were not diabetic, but whose bodies were producing too much insulin. He discovered that these patients had very low blood sugar levels. Dr. Harris devised a diet to help correct the disorder.

The body runs on sugar (blood glucose). The nervous system and brain must have a continual supply of glucose. It is the only source of energy for the brain. The body was designed to prevent blood sugar levels from plunging too low. However it was not designed to handle sudden changes in glucose levels, such as those caused by the over-consumption of refined sugar. The typical American diet is loaded with sugar. The sugar consumption starts for the child during the mothers pregnancy and lasts until death.

A normal person can eat a simple refined carbohydrate, such as white sugar and the blood level of sugar rises. Then the pancreas secretes the hormone insulin which soon brings down blood sugar to the fasting level. The hypoglycemic person can eat the same amount of white sugar and this puts the pancreas in shock which over-reacts secreting so much insulin into the blood that sugar is removed too rapidly, creating a glucose deficit.

Hypoglycemia is seen as the first step on the road to chronic degenerative disease because of its devastating effect on the body, especially in the stress related adrenals. When one gland is weakened it has an affect on all the glands. It has a wear and tear effect on the body. It affects the nervous system, muscles, cells as well as all the glands. Dr.

Robert Atkins, one of the foremost pioneers in the field of blood sugar disturbances says, "without improper nutrition, I don't believe diabetes could develop, even if both parents are diabetic. No one is doomed by heredity to develop diabetes." I feel that we are not doomed to develop hypoglycemia or many of the diseases plagued by mankind, just because our parents have it.

Hypoglycemia should be taken seriously, and corrected as soon as possible. It can cause serious problems, and is a forerunner of diabetes and Addison's disease. It can lead to other diseases such as cancer and heart disease. Hypoglycemia is an abnormal and potentially dangerous condition since reduced supplies of glucose to the brain can result in brain dysfunction and may lead to permanent cell damage. The brain requires a small but steady glucose supply and reacts immediately when it's ration is not supplied. This has an enormous impact on the personality. Brain starvation, from lack of steady flow of glucose to the brain brings on all kinds of unnatural symptoms.

The symptoms of hypoglycemia are very subtle to the person who has it. I have observed many people with hypoglycemia and their actions become so normal to them that they do not realize they are actng in a very negative and unusual way. Their way of perceiving and reacting to situations becomes distorted. One friend of mine went through a very traumatic period in her life. She knew that if she divorced her husband all her problems would be solved. Later when she was able to get her hypoglycemia under control, she realized that it wasn't her husband at all, it was her that was creating the problems.

A multitude of symptoms are caused when the body's glucose goes down. The brain shuts down the emergency compensator mechanism trying to get the glucose up again. The lack of fuel causes a dysfunction in the central nervous system and various disorders develop into symptoms of hypoglycemia.

SYMPTOMS OF HYPOGLYCEMIA

The best known symptom is fatigue. A fatigue not from good old fashioned hard work or exercise, which can create a rejuvenating and relaxing effect, but fatigue that pulls on all the muscles and nerves. A fatigue that sleep and rest never fully satisfy.

The symptoms are varied. Hypoglycemia can mimic many diseases.

2

Some doctors see the symptoms as a sign of neurosis, all in the mind and send their patients home with tranquilizers or send them to psychiatrists. These doctors feel that their waiting rooms were full of people who were really sick. A majority of symptoms involve the central nervous system. The body needs nerve food. The nervine herbs will restore and nourish the nervous system faster than any other food.

Low blood sugar levels affect every system of the body, and any symptom can result from hypoglycemia. That is why there are so many symptoms associated with hypoglycemia. Most people can experience many of these symptoms at one time or another. But the symptoms will not linger or reappear constantly. If the adrenal glands and pancreas are working properly the body chemistry is restored to normal and symptoms are relieved.

If hypoglycemia is actually the problem the symptoms may change to another set of symptoms. They may go away for a while but will soon reappear.

Amnesia
Anxiety
Antisocial Behavior
Breathing Difficulties
Confusion
Constant Worry
Crying Jags
Depression
Digestive Disorders
Dizziness
Drowsiness
Emotional Instability
Exhaustion
Fainting
Headaches
Heart Palpitation

Impatience
Inability to Cope
Insomnia
Intense Hunger
Internal Trembling
Irritability
Lack of Concentration
Nervousness
Numbness
Phobias (unjustified fears)
Seizures
Severe Sweating
Sugar Craving
Suicidal Tendencies
Tingling
Tremors

HYPOGLYCEMIA AND PANIC ATTACKS

Case History

Darla's story is a vivid illustration of the frightening reality of the experiences some can have that are now being referred to as panic attacks. Dr. Harold N. Levinson, M.D. refers to a panic attack as an individual experiencing a loss of control in the absence of any visible trigger. In Dr. Levinson's book, *Phobia Free,* he explores the idea that 90% of all phobias and panic attacks can be traced to a hidden physical problem.

Darla's story is a testimony to that. Darla experienced her first attack in the summer of 1985. She describes it as "feeling my blood running in my veins, a crawly feeling."

She had just undergone nose surgery and assumed that she may have been having a reaction to the drugs that she had been given during her surgery. She asked the doctor if this would be the case, but he was not sure.

The following year was a very stressful one for Darla. She lost her business and her home. In February of 1986 she began to experience that "crawly" feeling again. She didn't think much about it until one day she went with her daughter to the mall to look for a prom dress. When she entered the mall she began to feel "light headed and spacy". She thought that maybe she was weak and needed to eat something. She got some soup, but was feeling so spacy that she couldn't eat. She felt her "ears ringing" and it seemed as though she was "talking in a barrel." Her daughter was frightened to see her mom like this. Darla remembered a friend of hers who was into health, suggesting to her that a good remedy for low blood sugar levels was to drink some water with honey in it. The restaurant had no honey, so Darla found a health food store and within 15 to 20 seconds after taking the honey and water she snapped completely out of it. But she was pretty shaken up by what had occurred.

The attacks started to come more frequently and they were more severe. Darla relates, "my ears would shut off, and I would get that crawly feeling accompanied by a shortnees of breath and numbness in my feet and hands. I would be shaking inside."

She became fearful of having an attack. She would have them several

4

times in the day and night. They seemed so unpredictable. She had never had any problems with hypoglycemia or low blood sugar before, so she wasn't sure if that was related to her problem or not. One doctor suggested that she was having a nervous breakdown and needed to learn to relax. Darla had seen two of her aunts suffer from a nervous breakdown who were still struggling to recover and were on extensive drug therapy. Darla felt strongly that this was not what was happening to her. But the attacks went on for two months. She lost 20 pounds and became very depressed. She gave up her church job and began to wonder if she she was going crazy. She was afraid to go anywhere for fear of having an attack. She felt so out of control. She wondered if these attacks were life threatening. Her most severe attacks occurred in the movie theatre, grocery store, mall, and church. She felt desperate. No one seemed to know what was wrong.

Darla heard about a doctor who was also into a Holistic approach to health. She had always been interested in natural health and herbs and vitamins. In her first visit with this doctor she was diagnosed as having hypoglycemia brought on by the stress of surgery and losing her home and business. She learned that it is common for hypoglycemia to be brought on by a major stress--surgery, childbirth, divorce, or death in the family, etc. Her doctor taught her first how to control her hypoglycemia by eating more frequently (at least every two hours). She learned that she would bring her blood sugar level up quickly with diluted juice or seeds and nuts. (The honey was too sweet for her hypoglycemia condition). She would carry a can of pineapple juice and if she felt an attack coming on she could control it by drinking the juice. Darla's confidence increased as she learned that she could control these attacks. She became very successful at controlling the attacks. She started to become stronger and experienced wellness. And then she discovered what seem to her to be a very strange occurence. When she would return to the places where she had experienced a previous attack, she found that the memory of the attacks created such anxiety in her that she was bringing on the same symptoms of the original attacks. She knew in her mind why the attacks were caused and she knew she had the means to control them, but the anxiety upon being in the same enviornment in which she had experienced attacks before was so great that she seemed to lose the control she had worked so hard to find. She was discouraged. She was no fun to be around. She didn't want to go anywhere. She saw a show on T.V. which was on panic attacks and realized that this was a common phenomena.

Her holistic doctor had moved out of state so Darla looked for a counselor. For two years her counselor helped her not to be afraid of having an attack. The movie theatre seemed to be the hardest place. Many times she would have to leave because she could not breathe. She was taught deep breathing techniques. She learned to psych herself up before going into those places. She learned how to "talk" herself out of an attack. The process of daily meditation helped her to feel in control. The control she had worked so hard to find.

Today Darla feels that she is in control of her life. She still carries a can of pineapple juice in her purse for security measures. And she has learned to watch for warning signals.

She knows if she gets overstressed or over tired she can begin to experience a shortness of breath. She knows that this is a signal to slow down and stop trying to do everything and to try to be more consistent with her daily meditation. Darla relates. "I know now that I'll be OK. I hope that by sharing my experience others can be helped. Even if your problem doesn't seem to have a physical cause, I know the mind has a great power on the body. It can be controlled with time, patience, and a very willing spirit. We can control our lives and what happens to us."

Dr. Levinson relates that physical causes for panic attacks can be related to chemical imbalance, sharp fluctuation in hormone levels, some other shift in the chemical balance of the brain, and those things which cause CVS disorders (cerebellar-vestibular system), problems that affect the inner-ear system or processing center of the brain.

DARLA'S SUPPLEMENTS AND DIET

Darla drank **licorice** tea to strengthen the adrenals. It helped increase the effectivness of glucocorticoids (adrenal hormones) found in the liver. She took **dulse** to help control thyroid by supplying natural iodine. It helps regulate metabolism and helps all the glands to function properly. **Dulse** also helps to eliminate waste material and nourishes the blood with essential minerals. She took **CAYENNE** to help regulate circulation. It also helped her digestion, which was poor. It cleans the blood and increases the power of other herbs she was taking. She took **DONG QUAI** to help balance hormones. It relaxes the nerves and strengthens all internal organs and muscles.

She took **EVENING PRIMROSE OIL** to help in her mood swings, which were anxiety, irritability, headaches and fluid retention. It contains GLA (gamma-linolenic acid), which is essential to glandular health to stimulate hormone-like properties. She used **GARLIC,** which supplies minerals and acts like a natural antibiotic. It dissolves cholesterol. It builds and protects the immune system. She took **LADY'S SLIPPER,** which was excellent for her nerves. It is good for hysteria and irritability, which she was plagued with. It is high in natural calcium, selenium and zinc, which she needed to build up her immune system. She also used **LOBELIA** to calm her nerves, strengthen her stomach, lungs and circulation. It has beneficial effect on the whole body. She used **SENNA TEA** to help lubricate her bowels. It increases the intestinal peristalic movements. She used it with **GINGER** to prevent cramping.

VITAMINS AND MINERALS

She took vitamin A, C, and E to build her immune system and protect further damage. She took B12, lecithin and pantothenic acid. She took a calcium supplement which was low in calcium and high in magnesium. She had trouble assimilating calcium and took boron supplements to help her assimilate calcium. She took manganese, chromium and potassium. She also took raw thyroid and raw adreneal supplements.

DARLA'S DAILY DIET

For breakfast she used a variety of choices. She used small amounts of fruit in season, an apple, ½ banana, an orange, slice of pineapple, ½ grapefruit, or 1 cup of fresh cherries, blueberries, raspberries or strawberries. One cup of yogurt or kefir or goats milk. She used nuts and seeds. She ground them and put them on her yogurt. Almonds, sunflower, pumpkin, sesame, chia or flaxseeds. She also used cottage cheese from the health food store.

Some mornings she ate a cup of sprouted grains or seeds and a glass of kefir, yogurt or goats milk. Another morning she would eat a cup of cooked cereal such as millet, buckwheat, brown rice or oats. She put butter or olive oil on her cereal. Some mornings she ate buckwheat pancakes with fresh applesauce, or one or two eggs soft boiled, with a slice of whole grain bread. Rye bread was high on her list.

For lunch she would have cooked millet, buckwheat, oats or 7-grain cereal. A glass of goat's milk, with cold pressed oil on cereal, or butter. Another lunch would be ½ avocado with a vegetable salad, and a fresh glass of vegetable juice. Another lunch would consist of freshly prepared vegetables, or steamed vegetables, such as zucchini, squash, green beans, peas, corn, etc., 1 slice of natural cheese, a slice of whole-grain bread with a pat of raw butter. She would also have a lunch of beans and corn tortillas with fresh tomatoes, onions, garlic and chili salsa. Another day for lunch she would eat ½ canned salmon, sardines, or tuna fish, with a salad.

For dinner she would have either salad, sprouts, cooked vegetables, soups, and a baked potato. Sometimes she would have fresh vegetable salad with a glass of goats milk, and a slice of whole grain bread. She would sometimes alternate with what she had for lunch.

SNACKS BETWEEN MEALS

She would have a green drink, fresh made vegetable juice or a handful of nuts or seeds.

LIVER FUNCTION IN HYPOGLYCEMIA

A sluggish liver is the most common cause of hypoglycemia. The lack of thyroid thyroxin creates a sluggish liver. The liver is our storage and filtering plant for the body, which releases food elements on demand when needed by the body. Starches are changed into a form of sugar, glycogen and release as the body needs energy-building materials. The liver performs about thirty duties every day. It acts as an incinerator for wastes, a central heating plant, circulating warmth all through the body by way of the blood vessels.

The liver is the vital link between nutrition and the mind. Nutrients coming from the intestinal tract, go to the liver, where they are processed before they are released in the blood stream. If the liver is functioning properly it filters out the toxins and makes sure the blood is supplied with an even flowing of sugar and other essential nutrients. This insures that the adrenals and the nervous system do not have to cope with "internal emergencies" which happens when too much or too little glucose enters the blood stream all at once.

The liver filters the blood and removes any wastes, toxins, contaminants which might damage the cells or disrupt proper function in the glandular system. It removes pesticides, insecticides, which can be absorbed with food as well as dead cells the body is continually sluffing off.

If the liver is not functioning properly many of the toxins remain in the blood and circulate throughout the body. This affects the nervous system and the brain and creates apathy, depression and lethargy. This is the reason that there are many symptoms associated with hypoglycemia.

Excellent herbs for cleansing the liver are: Dandelion root, Golden Seal, Red Beet, Yellow Dock, Bayberry, Oregon Grape and Lobelia. parsley, Horsetail, Liverwort, Gentian, and Golden Rod are also excellent.

Pau D'Arco will purify the blood and liver. Red Clover is a blood purifier and liver cleanse. Ecninacea cleans the glands and liver.

Supplements to help the liver: Chlorophyll, lecithin, bentonite cleanse, Evening Primrose Oil, Fresh lemon and pure water, Fish oil, Garlic, and Glucomannan.

CAUSES OF HYPOGLYCEMIA

There are several causes of hypoglycemia which stem from a diet high in refined food and excessive sugar intake. Causes include: Stress, Glandular dysfunction and mineral deficiencies. The typical American diet is high in processed food, food chemically treated, overcooked, stripped of nutrients, sweetened and salted and altered in many ways. Fried foods are a typical diet that disrupt the glandular system.

Processed food contains a great amount of sucrose, which contributes to hypoglycemia. The hidden sugar in food means that if we eat a normal American diet we consume hundreds of pounds of sucrose (white sugar) every year.

Sugar is added to food products to increase consumption. Sugar is a very addictive substance; the low blood sugar state which you get from eating it makes you crave more. The food industry have discovered that increasing the sugar in a product also increases the amount a person will eat, which will increase sales.

High sugar intake wears on the glandular system, which can lose its ability to regulate the metabolism of carbohydrates and thus keep the brain properly nourished with glucose. Sugar is stripped of vital nutrients which contribute to mental disorders. White sugar is not a food, it is a chemical.

STRESS

Stress, (both physical and mental) is a major factor in hypoglycemia. It is a vicious cycle which is difficult to escape...Anxiety can induce low blood sugar and low blood sugar causes anxiety. Worry and strife upset the endocrine balance, which then contributes to underproduction of blood glucose. Stress weakens our immune system and causes the overproduction of toxins called free radicals which causes cell damage. Stress seriously affects body chemistry and the glands. We burn nutrients at a tremendous pace when we are under constant stress.

Stress is manifested everyday in one form or another. We are exposed to **CHEMICAL STRESS** in the form of pesticides, insecticides, heavy metals, asbestos, polluted air, polluted water and radioactive wastes. Drugs of all kinds put a heavy burden on the body.

EMOTIONAL STRESS hits us when we have to face life style changes. It can be a good change or a bad change, either one puts extra stress on the body. It comes in the form of marriage, divorce, death in the family, new baby, change of job, moving, etc.

PHYSICAL STRESS puts an extra stress on the nervous system as well as the body. It can come in the form of a car accident, broken bones, sport accident, burns, cuts, bruises, illness of any kind. Illness puts a burden on the organs of the body and weakens the immune system. This comes in the form of colds, flu, and an acute disease that can weaken the body more if surpressed by drugs and eating wrong foods, which stops the natural course of an actue disease.

Chronic or extreme stress puts a burden on the liver which stores glycogen and prevents it from providing sufficient amounts to maintain adequate glucose levels in the blood and hypoglycemia results.

Stressful stiuations over months and years depleted resources of the pancreas and adrenal glands which come to the rescue under "emergency reactions".

Stress activates hormone production. A normal body, under stress will produce two main hormones from the adrenal gland. These hormones are cortin, which is the "stress-coping" hormone, and adrenalin, which is the fight or flight hormone. Over a period of time, ongoing stress, (in a short period of time, if the stress is great), the adrenals become worn out and cannot produce an adequate amount of the hormones. Dietary "stress" affects the body virtually the same way. Sugars that the body doesn't need right away are stored as glycogen in the liver and muscles. When the body is under stress, the release of adrenalin, stimulates the breakdown of glycogen into glucose. Frequent releases of adrenalin will exhaust the adrenal glands, so that adrenalin is no longer produced. Hence, the blood sugar levels are not maintained at a balanced level and the person will crave sweets to bring up the blood sugar, which dips to a dangerous low when glycogen is not supplied.

In order to lower the stress factor the nervous system needs to be taken care of first. It needs to be strengthened along with the immune system. This will help the body cope with stress and prevent further complications.

GLANDULAR DYSFUNCTION: When a person eats a lot of refined carbohydrates, it affects the entire endocrine or glandular system. The hypothalamus alerts the pituitary to release a hormone which raises the blood sugar level. This, in turn, stimulates the adrenal gland, to produce the stress hormones, which in turn, temporarily lower the blood sugar.

The thyroid gland controls the rate at which the blood sugar is burned and the pancreas is responsible for controlling the blood glucose level. The liver manufactures a substance called glycogen from the excess blood sugar and stores it for times of need, when the body requires glucose. When this delicate interaction between the glands is disturbed, it is known as "glandular dysfunction". The blood sugar levels are not kept at an even balance and abnormal blood sugar or inadequate blood sugar levels will ensue, depending on which gland is affected. If the adrenals are exhausted, it will manifest itself as low blood sugar, or HYPOGLYCEMIA. If the pancreas is stressed out, it will show up as high blood sugar, or DIABETES. Wildly fluctuating blood sugar levels wreak havoc upon the entire endocrine system. When there is an excessive intake of refined carbohydrates, it causes a rapid rise in blood sugar. Hypoglycemics are very sensitive to rises in the blood sugar. In these individuals the pancreas overreacts by secreting very high levels of insulin. The adrenals then produce adrenalin which stimulates the liver to break down stored forms of glucose, or glycogen. It is released into the bloodstream as glucose, to compensate for the lowered blood sugar levels. Soon the adrenals are exhausted and cannot help in the conversion. The body signals for help to assist in raising the blood sugar. The person craves a sugary substance and the yo-yo syndrome continues. The mental and physical state of the hypoglycemic then deteriorates further. The vicious cycle is perpetuated. Consequently, when the adrenals become exhausted and the person eats sweet foods to get a rise in energy, the pancreas is called upon more and more to produce insulin. This is why in many cases, doctors tell their patients that their hypoglycemia can eventually turn into diabetes. Once the pancreas cannot produce any more insulin, the person is in a serious medical condition.

MINERAL DEFICIENCIES: Sugar or (sucrose) contributes to an imbalance in the body. It creates stress by leaching the vitamin B complex and calcium which causes an imbalance in calcium, potassium, magnesium and sodium in the body. Dr. William J. Goldwag says, "chemical imbalance is not a specific disease. It refers to any condition or set of circumstances which changes the normal pattern of chemical rections in the body." He says, "the body does not tolerate imbalance for more than a brief instant before it goes into action with various chemical changes designed to protect and preserve us in the way it has learned best. This produces a new state of balance to suit the new conditions. We may not like the new state of balance because it may cause us unpleasant symptoms, but remember, the body is doing its best to adjust its chemistry. If we wish to change the situation and get rid of symptoms or heal, we must activate chemical responses that adjust conditions back to a more desirable kind of balance." Nutrition can play a vital role in supplying the necessary nutrients in the amounts and in the areas of the body where they are needed so the body can do its own re-balancing act in accordance with our aims of health and high energy.

It has been discovered that a lack of certain essential minerals necessary in helping with conversion of glycogen to glucose, can also promote low blood sugar. One of these essential nutrients is Chromium. The trace mineral chromium transports glucose from the blood into the cells, thus increasing the effectiveness of insulin. A compound, containing chromium, was discovered in the late 1960's. It was named the Glucose Tolerance Factor. It consists of chromium complexed from niacin and glutathione (glutamic acid, glycine and cystine). Maximum absorption of chromium is realized in this form, as opposed to straight chromium supplementation. GTF chromium is said to reduce symptoms of hypoglycemia such as fatigue, irritability, hunger, and headaches, by controlling insulin production. GTF uses the existing circulating insulin to maintain optimal levels of blood sugar. When white sugar products are ingested, the sucrose bypasses the normal glycogen-conversion, wherein the body converts glucose for the blood as it is needed. The pure sucrose goes directly to the blood stream, full force and touches off abnormally high insulin-production. If the adrenals are exhausted and cannot help with matching glycogen-glucose production, then the person could go into "insulin shock". This is manifested by faintness, hunger, heart palpitations and sweating. Sometimes the individual can appear to be intoxicated. Glucose is the only form of energy that the brain can "burn", except for glutamic acid (and amino acid). A combination of glucose and oxygen keeps our brains functioning. If a person is deficient in vitamin B1 (thiamine) the glucose cannot be burned for energy, once it reaches the brain. Glucose is not stored in brain tissue, so the only way the brain can be healthy is if blood glucose remains at an adequate steady level. Consequently, low blood sugar can contribute to emotional disturbances and mental disorders.

REFINED FOODS

In the book *Body, Mind and The B Vitamins,* the authors point out: "Nature likes things whole. Nothing worthwhile is achieved in nature with fragments. Lifting all of the B-complex vitamins from our wholegrain cereals...when they are milled and processed...then returning only bits of three of the B vitamins synthetically is probably the worst possible thing we could do, for the imbalances thus created are unimaginably complex. Many of the trace minerals are also lost in this refining process...As you add white sugar and foods made from it, you cut down severely on the vitmain B content of your diet, for all vitamins have been removed from the sugar cane to make white sugar. You also create imbalances because Nature has arranged that the B vitamins are essential for the body to process starches and sugars...There is a close relation between the amount of pyridoxine (B6) and fluctuations of blood sugar, indicating that deficiency in this vitamin may have something to do with both diabetes and low blood sugar."

A diet high in sugars and starches has been shown to deplete the body of B vitamins. B vitamin deficiency has been linked to depression, PMS, and fatigue as well as many other ailments. Richard J. Walsh states in the book *Treating Your Hyperactive and Learning Disabled Child,* "Blood tests reveal that 75 percent of hyperactive, learning disabled children have hypoglycemia and/or allergies. These disorders indicate stress in the body and affect the visual function of a child...Our observations...indicate sugar as a critcal culprit in producing symptoms of hyperactivity and learning disorders...the majority of these children eat a high percentage of concentrated sweets. Most have difficulty metabolizing carbohydrates..."

GLANDULAR SYSTEM AND RAW FOOD

Raw foods are necessary for the glandular system. Cooked food kills the enzymes and causes the endocrine glands to become overworked and leads to body intoxication and diseases such as hypoglycemia, diabetes and obesity.

Cooked foods over stimulate the glands and cause the body to retain excess weight. The enzymes from live food help the body to maintain proper metabolism.

The problem arises when the glands do not receive the nutrients necessary to satisfy the body's needs. When this happens the glands overstimulate the digestive organs and demand more food (because the body is not satisfied). This produces an oversecretion of hormones, an unhealthy appetite, which finally results in exhaustion of the hormone-producing glands.

ENDOCRINE (GLANDULAR) FUNCTION AND HYPOGLYCEMIA

The endocrine glands secrete hormones for full body activity directly into the blood stream. The glands are so vital for our over all health that nature protects them by placing them in areas of the body where they are protected by bony tissues and membranes. The glands of the body are the officers and/or leaders of body emotions and functions. The glands get their orders directly form the brain and spinal cord and have life and death control of the entire body. It is essential that we keep these glands healthy, with the finest nutrition possible. It is important and vital that the blood stream be pure and that the veins and arteries be clear and free of fatty deposits. The blood must be flowing freely and the heart functioning normally to get pure blood to all the glandular areas at all times if we expect excellent mental and physical health.

Scientists used to believe that the brain was insulated from the rest of the body by the blood/brain barrier, and that diet did not have much to do with a healthy endocrine system. A major breakthrough occured when Dr. Richard J. Wurtman and his colleagues at the Massachusetts Institute of Technology demonstrated that diet does contain precursors of brain neurotransmiters which modulate aspects of mood, mind, memory and behavior.

Dr. Wurtman has demonstrated in his research that carbohydrates in a meal stimulate the production of insulin which, it turn, facilitates the uptake of the amino acid tryptophan across the blood/brain barrier. Tryptophan is then used by specific regions of the brain for the synthesis and secretion of the neurotransmitter serotonin, which has a calming effect upon mood.

We know that an iodine deficiency has an impact on the thyroid and can produce goiter. Recent studies have demonstrated that zinc insufficiency may have an adverse impact upon thymus secretion of the hormone thymosin which, in turn, has a T-lymphocyte regulatory effect.

Nutrition also has an impact upon the behavior mechanisms of the hypothalamus and pituitary. Animal studies over the past several years have shown that marginal deprivation of certain nutrients and calories can result in suppression of normal appetite mechanisms in the hypothalamus, resulting in eating disorders. This may put a new light on eating disorders as anorexia nervosa, bulimia and compulsive eating, and the effect the lack of nutrients has on the endocrine and nervous systems.

Proper nutrition does have an impact on a healthy endocrine system.

Each gland plays an important role to overall health of the whole body. When one gland isn't working properly it can affect other glands. It is important that we understand the glands and the nutrients that will clean, build and strengthen them.

PITUITARY GLAND

The pituitary gland is attached to the hypothalamus at the base of the brain. This area of the brain controls almost all body functions through a network of releasing factors and hormones which control the rate of growth, metabolic rate, electrolyte balance, ovulation and lactation. The hypothalamus secretes peptide releasing factors to the pituitary which secretes more peptide hormones into the bloodstream to control the function of the entire endocrine system.

The pituitary is called the master gland because it affects the entire endocrine (glandular) system. It is a gland that should be strengthened and nourished properly because of its function with any gland such as thyroid, adrenal or pancreas and for inblances of the sex glands and poor maturation of secondary sex traits. Its use would also be indicated in high stress and in conditions of hypoglycemia.

Pituitary hormones help to maintain water balance. It has an influence on kidney function. A very weak pituitary causes frequent urination, swollen ankles, bags under the eyes, and a general bloated appearance. It is estimated that 88% of women have underactive pituitary glands. If the anterior portion of the pituitary is strong instead of weak, it will upset body chemistry and result in moon face, fat on back of neck, excess weight on trunk while arms and legs stay slender.

The growth-monitoring portion of the pituitary gland contains 7 to 10 times the bromine concentration of any other organ. Kelp and dulse contain traces of bromine, as do mussles, sea water and animal glands.

Lack of potassium and sodium can cause pituitary inbalance. Potassium herbs are: Dulse, irish moss, valerian, stevia, scullcap, saffron, red clover, parsley, licorice, horsetail, hops and garlic. Sodium herbs are: Alfalfa, chickweed, buchu, burdock, gotu kola, saffron, sarsaparilla, rosehips, parsley, licorice and dandelion. An herbal combination to balance endocrine system: Kelp, irish moss, parsley, hops and capsicum. Mullein and lobelia are also good. Suma, a new herb from Brazil has been known to help the glands.

The blood needs to be cleaned. A red clover blend, chaparral, pau d'arco are excellent. Golden seal and echinacea are also excellent.

All glands need iodine and silicon. Iodine is found in kelp and dulse. Silicon is found in horsetail or oatstraw.

Vitamin E is essential for all the glands. B complex vitamins with extra B6. Vitamin A and C are also essential. Amino acids for pituitary are: Ornithine, tryptophan, and taurine. Arginne and lysine nourish the pituitary.

Sprouts: Aflafla, buckwheat, radish and fenugreek are benefical for the glands.

Dr. John Ott suggests that the light coming through the eyes reacts on the pituitary glands. This gland being the master gland reacts on all the other glands in the body.

ADRENAL GLANDS

The adrenal glands are located on top of the kidneys, approximately at the middle of the back, where they are protected by the spine and muscular structure. They manufacture steroids, which are sex hormones, indispensable to life. The adrenals secrete fight or flight hormones which relieve stressful situations by increasing heart beat, raising blood sugar, adding to oxygen output and heat consumption and aiding muscles by stimulating the body power levels to cope with physical emergencies.

The adrenal cortex produces three groups of hormones in response to stimulation from pituitary hormones. One group of hormones stimulates the retention of sodium in the body and the excretion of potassium. The second group of hormones affects glucose, amino acids and fat metabolism. The steroid hormones in this group help to maintain a steady supply of essential building blocks and fuel to maintain normal body repair and growth in all tissues. These hormones are also involved in the control of inflammation in the body. The third group of hormones are the sex hormones, both male and female hormones.

Adrenalin is highly poisonous when secreted in excess and affects the whole system. When the adrenals are not working properly and producing hormones the body collects and retains toxic waste in the lymphatic system. Red Clover and Echinacea will help the lymphatics.

Tobacco smoke contains two irritating poisons nicotine and acrolein.

Inhaling this smoke stimulates an excessive secretion of adrenalin. These poisons are collected from the mouth way down to the bottom of the lungs by the lymph stream. This builds up and weakens the lungs and the adrenals.

Mullein and lobelia are perfect glandular foods. Siberian Ginseng strengthens the whole body as well as the glands. Gotu Kola stimulates brain and relieves fatigue. Hawthorn Berries strengthen heart when under stress. Cayenne aids in circulation of blood, which brings oxygen and other nutrients to cells in need or repair. Ginger stimulates blood and cleans capillaries.

Licorice root is food for the adrenal glands. It acts like cortisone and steroids. Cortisone is a steroid sugar. Licorice does not act like sugar, even though it is three times as sweet. Wild yam also acts like cortisone.

Saffron helps the body to use oils which protect the gall bladder and liver. It allows the body to regulate lactic acid, and prevents aching joints. Aching joints are one of the first signs that the adrenals are exhausted. The adrenals are too exhausted to produce the hormones that prevent pain and inflammation.

Fear and resentment wear out the adrenal glands.

To strengthen the adrenals blend together the following and soak in pure water overnight. Eat throughout the day. One half cup ground almonds, two tablespoons each of sunflower seeds, pumpkin and sesame. One tablespoon of flax and chia seeds. Put in a container and cover with water. Be ready to eat the next morning.

Vitamin C with bioflavinoids are concentrated in the adrenal glands, it is depleted fast when under stress or illness. Vitamin A repairs damaged tissues. Zinc cleans and repairs tissues. Evening primrose oil helps adrenals.

THYMUS

The thymus gland is located under the sternum (breast bone) and it is part of the lymph system. It is related to sexual activity and functions in stressful situations. It atrophies early when not cared for or when abused with additives, drugs, alcohol, nicotine and inadequate nutrients.

During the adolescence period the thymus acts as a balance between higher and lower instincts. The thymus actually influences a person's character. Dr. N.W. Walker, D. Sc., says, "If an adolescent is allowed to go about his way of life unbridled, undisciplines and uncontrolled, the thymus gland will become flabby in texture and in years to come he will find himself on the lower, if not the lowest, plane of consciousness. At this period in life the thymus works in close relation with the pineal gland, the spiritual gland, children of all ages need affection and understanding, as well as the right kind of nourishment."

The thymus gland will actually shrivel under stress. The thymus controls the energy flow throughout the body. The thymus is the first organ of the body to feel the impact of stressful situations. It is also affected by the emotional state of the mind. The thymus is also influenced by the physical environment of individuals and the food they eat, their posture, and relationships with others. The thymus is more sensitive to nutritional deficits than most other organs and protein-energy malnutrition has a very profound effect on the body, and especially on the thymus. The thymus releases hormones that creat age-fighting lymphocytes, which are white blood cells that produce antibodies to fight off infectious bacteria and diseases.

Vitamin A and zinc are needed to keep the thymus functioning properly. Vitamin C is the most important nutrient in the health of all the glands. B-complex vitamins are specific for the thymus. Vitamin A, C, E, and B-complex are synergistic to the thymus in increasing immunity. Zinc, manganese, copper and iron are also important as coenzymes for the synthesis of protein and as active agents in destroying many toxins.

PANCREAS

The pancreas has two important functions in the body. 1. Secreting digestive enzymes to break down protein, fat and carbohydrate in the duodenum, and 2. neutralizing the highly acidic juices from the stomach and regulating glucose.

The endocrine function of the pancreas is carried out by specialized tissues called the islets of Langerhans, which secrete the hormones insulin and glucagon into the bloodstream. Both hormones are important in controlling the level of blood sugar in the body. It is important to control the blood glucose levels, it is the only nutrient that can be utilized by the brain, retina, and germinal epithelium.

19

The pancreas doesn't work alone, it is assisted by all the other glands.

The following herbal combination was formulated to heal all the glands. Cedar berries, licorice root, uva ursi, golden seal root, mullein, and capsicum.

The cedar berries are food for the pancreas and help in kidney and bladder problems. Licorice root is a glandular food and cleanser. All of the glands will benefit and be nourished with licorice. Uva ursi is an excellent herb for the adrenal, it stimulates digestion and helps control obesity. It assists in controlling kidney and bladder congestion. Golden seal is excellent antiseptic and cleanser for the glandular system, it heals digestive problems. Mullein is a specific herb for the glandular system and it cleans and rebuilds all of the glands and supplies minerals. Capsicum aids the pancreas, digestive system and all the glands. It stimulates the circulation for rapid healing.

The pancreas manufactures enzymes which are passed through a duct into the digestive system. 1. Pacreactic lipase which acts upon fats that have already been emulsified by bile and transform them into fatty acids and glycerol, a fatty substance. Fatty acids are necessary to provide a concentrated source of calories for energy. Fats also aid in storage and assimilation of vitamins A, D, E, and K. Fats are also necessary to aid in certain processes of metabolism and cell structure. Fatty acids build the structure of the brain and nerve tissues. 2. Trypsin is a pancreatic enzyme which acts upon proteins; particularly those which have not been partially digested in the stomach. It also acts upon the foods that have been partially treated by pepsin, breaking down these substances into peptides. 3. Amylase, serves to split uncooked as well as cooked starch into maltose, a substance that can be utilized by the body.

NUTRITIONAL SUPPLEMENTS FOR PANCREAS

Vitamin A - essential for all the mucus membranes, promotes healing in all the glands.

B-Complex - helps combat stress. Extra pantothenic acid helps to normalize sugar levels. B6 is needed to prevent damage to the pancreas.

Vitamin C - helps to normalize sugar metabolism, and strengthens the body's ability to tolerate sugar and carbohydrate. Protects the immune system.

Vitamin E - protects the glands from destruction by increasing oxygen. Improves the oxygenation of the cells.

Mineral Balanced Supplement - Manganese deficiency can cause pancreas problems. Sulphur strengthens the pancreas and protects against infections. Selenium provides protection of oxidation of cell membranes.

HYPOTHALAMUS

The hypothalamus is located at the base of the brain. It transmits and receives brain messages to and from every other part of the body. It is considered part of the brain and controls many essential involuntary human functions, such as blood pressure, heart rate and body temperature. It controls the secretion of hormones by the anterior pituitary. It is best known for its key role in the control of appetite and satiety.

The hypothalamus records memory. If you have ever had food creavings when on a cleansing program (and who hasn't) the hypothalamus helps you remember what it used to taste like. Memory plays a major role in cravings.

It affects the storage of fat, weight set point, movement, the senses and a variety of other important behavioral and physical functions.

The hypothalamus stimulates the pituitary gland which in turn stimulates the adrenal gland to produce cortisone-like substances. All the glands need to be kept in tip top shape, they are all interrelated.

Gotu Kola - A brain food. Helps balance hormones and relaxes the nerves and combats stress.

Co Q10 - Protects the body against free radicals.

Germanium - Increases oxygen in the blood to protect the body.

Suma - Contains germanium, which protects the immune system.

Balances hormone for both men and women.

Burdock - blood purifier, stimulates and nourishes the hypothalamus.

Minerals - Zinc helps in eating disorders such as anorexia and bulimia. Necessary for normal hypothalamic function.

Amino Acids - L-arginine, L-phenylalanine. Tryptophan is the enzymatic precursor to the brain neurotransmitter serotonin. Helps curb cravings.

PINEAL GLAND

The pineal gland is shaped like a pine cone and is located at the base of the brain behind and above the pituitary gland. It works with the pituitary to play a major role in reproduction, growth, body temperature, blood pressure, motor activity, sleep and mood.

In ancient times it was called "seat of the soul". The pineal gland is associated with spirituality and is involved with the pituitary gland. It is in cooperation with the pituitary gland in brain function, such as reason, judgement, memory, reflection, love, worship, etc.

It is an important gland that acts like radar. Some scientists feel that the pineal gland along with the pituitary anticipates environmental flucuations and prepares the animal for temperature changes, reproduction, activity, rest and hibernation. This gland is regulated by environmental light and the earth's electromagnetic field. Its activity is affected by the amount of available light it receives through the retina of the eye and by the electromagnetic field of the earth. The dark winter months can produce depression, weight gain and lethargy. Light therapy has proven effective in seasonal depression.

The pineal gland may play a role in some diseases such as cancer, heart disease, Parkinson's disease and Alzheimers disease. One study reported that the hormone melatonin was administrated to Parkinson patients and resulted in reduced symptoms of tremor and rigidity, which may suggest that the hormone may also play a role in brain electrical activity.

The pineal gland which secretes the hormone melatonin during periods of darkness, suppresses that hormone in the presence of bright light. Melatonin can have adverse emotional mental and physical effects. Insomnia, increased appetite, irritation, sadness and fatigue are some of the adverse effects. Indoor lighting is not sufficient enough to suppress melatonin. This explains why there are more people depressed in the winter months. Vitamin A and beta-carotene is quickly used up when we are in the sun. It is a protection. Vitamin A is important to the proper functioning of the pineal gland protecting its photoreceptor cells from damage.

GONADS

The gonads are the sexual endocrine glands. Sexual hormones are released from the hypothalamus and the pituitary in both the female and male. The gonadal glands in the male are the testes. A variety of male sex hormones are produced in the testes, the most potent and abundant is testosterone. This hormone promotes primary and secondary male sexual characteristics.

Testosterone is responsible for many metabolic changes. At puberty testosterone increases and causes hair growth, enlargement of sexual organs, and larynx (results in deeper voice), increased muscular development and bone size and strength.

The ovaries are the female gonadal glands. The ovaries produce estrogen and progesterone according to the monthly cycle. Extrogen is responsible for most female secondary sexual characteristics. It causes breast development, increased bone and protein deposition, stimulates hair growth on pubis and arm-pits, and thicker skin.

Progesterone prepares the uterus for pregnancy and the breasts for lactation. Progesterone is secreted in the last half of the ovaries cycle and during pregnancy, in larger quantities by the placenta, estrogen is more potent than progesterone.

Vitamin E is specific to the sex glands, both male and female. A degeneration in the function of the sex glands synchronizes the gradual breakdown of the tissues which leads to senility.

Protein is essential, along with tryptophane, lysine, linoleic acid, Iron and Vitamins A, B, and C.

THYROID GLAND

The thyroid is a small butterfly-shaped gland in the neck, weighs less than an ounce, yet its hormone secretions control body metabolism, the way in which the body transforms foods and uses energy. Too much thyroid hormone-hyperthyroidism can race body processes and produce strain, weight loss, irritability. Too little-hypothyroidism can slow the processes, affecting both physical and mental activity.

The thyroid acts as an energizer and lubricator for an adult and helps in growth and development of tissues for a child. Approximately five quarts of blood circulate through the thyroid gland once every hour. The thyroid needs a constant supply of iodine in order to maintain the proper supply of thyroxine in the tissues.

Stephen E. Langer, M.D., author of *Solved: The Riddle of Illness,* says: "Inadequate thyroid function is an unsuspected contributer to a number of physical conditions, including elevated cholesterol levels and atherosclerosis, complications of diabetes, premenstrual syndrome and fertility problems."

"Most people with low thyroid tend to have high cholesterol and triglyceride levels, which go down generally anywhere from 10 to 20 percent without any change in their diet."

The drug Thalidomide depressed thyroid secretion as to result in failure of fetal cells to reproduce and multiply as a consequence, the baby is armless, legless or otherwise deformed.

Poor diet upsets body chemistry, skin eruptions, bulging eyes, unstable emotions, nervous energy and heavy perspiration. Lack of thyroxine hormones causes wasting tissues, nervous disorders, damaged teeth and muscles, skin and hair damage. Underactive thyroid causes slow circulation and the tissues become flabby.

A well functioning thyroid makes life worth while, exciting. It controls vitality, growth, and protects against poisons and injuries.

BASAL TEMPERATURE TEST FOR LOW THYROID

The best time for this test is immediately upon awakening in the morning. Before going to bed shake down a thormometer and place it on the bedside table. This test is taken before getting out of bed. Immediately upon awakening, place the thermometer snugly in the armpit for 10 minutes by the clock. The normal basal temperature is between 97.8 and 98.1 degrees. A temperature below 97.8 degrees indicates the possibility of low thyroid activity. FOR WOMEN: As the temperature varies with the phases of the menstrual cycle, the test should be made on the second and third days of menstruation. CHILDREN: In young children, rectal temperture can be taken; two minutes are adequate. Oral temperatures are often misleading, because any respiratory infection, including sinusitis, will elevate the mouth temperature while the rest of the body may be subnormal. (Hope for Hypoglycemia, by Broda O. Barnes, M.D., Ph.D. and Charlotte W. Barnes, A.M.)

Natural iodine is found in kelp, dulse, irish moss, watercress, black walnut and spirulina. Oatstraw tea helps to rejuvenate all the glands.

A vitamin supplement plus B-complex. Phenylalanin and tyrosine are vital for proper function of the thyroid.

Mineral supplement, calcium and magnesium. Zinc necessary for proper thyroid function.

PARATHYROIDS

The parathyroids are four glands attached to the thyroid. Their main function is to control and regulate the supply of calcium and vitamin D in the body. They have an influence over the lymph system in neutralizing toxins in the body.

A deficiency of the parathyroid creates a sensitivity of the nervous system. It creates a temperamental characteristc, and antisocial behavior. Calcium and vitamin D are essential. Alfalfa and kelp are specific herbs for the parathyroid glands.

HYPOGLYCEMIA AND CRIME

Hypoglycemia is a disorder characterized by irrational behavior, distorted judgement, emotional instability restlessness and ugly personality defects. These personality types have been linked to crime, alcohol and drug abuse. This type of anti-social behavior has been linked time and time again to lack of nutrients, caused by sugar-laden diets.

Sugar (sucrose) is a chemical. White table sugar has been refined, adulterated and denatured. It is stripped of all nutrients. It enters the bloodstream quickly. You can consume sugar faster than when it is in its natural state, (such as fruit). The body cannot use white sugar properly, it absorbs too rapidly. It enters into the bloodstream within minutes. The body needs a gradual rise in serum glucose, not the quick fix it gets with sugar.

We as Americans consume so much refined sucrose that our endocrine systems are in constant shock. The pancreas is overworked tyring to produce insulin as soon as it senses sugar in the blood. As blood sugar drops, the cerebrum, (the part of the brain responsible for thought, learning, and moral and social behavior) starts to slow down and reverses to primitive responses.

In order to digest white sugar the body must use its own supply of minerals and vitamins, which leads to imbalances and deficiencies in the body. This will eventually cause damage to the organs, brain and nervous system.

Prison, jails and detention centers have observed through studies a high rate of hypoglycemia among the inmates, averaging 80 to 85 percent. The problem is treated in most institutions as non-existent.

Barbara Ree, Ph.D., author of *Food, Teens and Behavior,* says, that "she is completely convinced that dietary therapy is one of the most powerful tools available for the treatment of emotional and behavioral disorders." Barbara is a probation officer and created a nutritional program which has helped thousands to lead healthy and productive lives. Eliminating white sugar was vital.

In her experience she says, "more than 80% of the probationers who have come to me since I started the orchomolecuor approach are living full productive lives today. Not a single individual who has stuck with the program has ever been in trouble with the law again."

ALCOHOLISM, DRUG ADDICTION AND HYPOGLYCEMIA

Hypoglycemia is common among drug addictors and alcoholics, they are notoious for their poor eating habits. Drugs such as heroin, methadon, tobacco and alcohol deplete the body's store of essential vitamins and minerals.

High sugar products are the staple ingredient in the diet of many addicts. Michael Smith of the Lincoln Detox Program suggest that the abnormally high rate of sugar consumption of narcotic addicts is due to several factors:

1). Intestinal spasm caused by narcotics makes digestion and absorption of more complex foods difficult.

2). Strain on liver caused by injected toxins leads to reduced food assimilation and glycogen storage function.

3). Addictive component of hypoglycemia which stems from the "sugar--over-reactive insulin--more sugar cycle."

4). Lack of concern for self-help common to addicts.

5). Intense marketing of sugar products, especially in poor communities. (*The Herbal Connection,* by Ethan Nebelkopf, M.A., M.F.C.C., page 40).

The B-complex vitamins are essential for a healthy nervous system. They are the "anti-stress" vitamins, which are destroyed by sugar, alcohol and drugs. Most addicts are deficient in B vitamins and this is reflected in their difficulty in dealing with stress.

Vitamin E protects against many enviornmental poisons in the air, food and water. Helps lower blood pressure and essential for the healthy functioning of the sex organs. Addicts and former addicts use vitamin E to heal many years of needle puncture on the legs, arms and skin surface. Vitamin E promotes healing of scar tissue. Aloe vera will also heal scar tissue, both inside the body and out.

Niacin helps to clean out impurities from the bloodstream. aids the circulation and inhibits the production of adrenalin. It aids in withdrawl from alcohol, barbiturates and heroin because of its anti-convulsant effects.

Vitamin C helps to overcome drug addiction.

Herbs to help detoxification of drugs. Comfrey, Mullein, Chaparral, Golden Seal and Rosehips. Herbs to strengthen the nerves: Lady's slipper, scullcap, hops, valerian root and passion flower. Herbs for energy: Suma, gotu kola, ginseng and sarsaparilla. Nutritional herbs: Alfalfa, dandelion, comfrey, horsetail, oatstraw, red clover, and yellow dock.

PMS AND HYPOGLYCEMIA

The reason many women crave sweets and chocolate just before their menstrual period is due to the drop in blood sugar, which is a temporary "hypoglycemia". Besides the sugar craving, some other symptoms blamed on this condition include fatigue, dizziness, and erratic behavior. Some forms of erratic behavior are: eating an entire box of candy at one sitting, food binges, and arguing without knowing why. This hypoglycemia is linked to shifts in the ratio between estrogen and progesterone. When there are elevated levels of estrogen in the body more insulin is released into the blood stream. This causes the drop in blood sugar.

High amounts of estrogen produce depression. When the diet is poor and the liver cannot eliminate the excess properly it goes back into the bloodstream and causes depression and other symptoms. When this is combined with the low blood sugar "blues" you have a compound case of severe depression or moodiness. One woman called her birth control pills her "grouch pills". Birth control pills containing high amounts of estrogen will accentuate the problem. Eating sugar to give oneself a "lift" from the low blood sugar "blues" will only make things worse. Sugar dissolves calcium out of the body, because it attracts calcium. Calcium is leached principally from the bones and teeth. B vitamins, which are essential to combat depression, are destroyed by high sugar intake. Increased irritability has been associated with ingestion of this devitalized substance. There are natural foods which will help restore the blood sugar balance in the body. (Further reading: **PMS: A Nutritional Approach**, by Louise Tenney).

MENTAL ILLNESS AND HYPOGLYCEMIA

Hypoglycemia is associated with mental illness. About one quarter of schizophrenics suffer from hypoglycemia, according to psychiatrists at the North Nassau Center, and "schizophrenic patients who have hypoglycemia cannot recover unless you correct it." Dr. Yaryura-Tobias says. (Other physicians estimate the rate of hypoglycemia among schizophrenics ist at around 60 percent).

In "Singing Low-Down Sugar Blues" by Joan Davidson, (12/81 issue of Chimo), she states: "Sugar addiction is a common factor in hypoglycemia; most people who suffer from this disease have a severe 'sweet tooth'. They crave sugar as an 'upper' because it increases their blood sugar levels and makes them feel less lethargic. Like drug addiction, this is a very real problem. Anyone who has been raised on refined sugar will feel deprived if they do not have sweets or starchy foods for even two or three days. And, like drug addiction, sugar addiction is very hard to kick. Sugar withdrawl symptoms include depression and anger and usually occur in a change in eating habits. The list of physical and mental problems which accompany hypoglycemia is almost unbelievable. Hypoglycemics experience a lack of energy, fatigue, or even complete exhaustion and fainting. Their symptoms have been described as: "...apathy, loss of zest, a general letdown feeling of aimlessness, a revulsion against the routine of everyday life, be it occupational activity of house hold duties." Chest, stomach, or severe back pains can also develop and disturbed sleep, insomnia and migraine headaches are quite common.

One study of mentally ill patients illustrates the dramatic effect a simple change in diet can have upon hypoglycemics. In this study 90% of 225 mentally ill patients (or 205 of them) were found to have hypoglycemia. In every case, their symptoms of mental illness desappeared only ten days after the implementation of a special diet which excluded, among other things, caffeine."

ALLERGIES AND HYPOGLYCEMIA

Hypoglycemia, celiac disease, multiple sclerosis, diabetes, epilepsy, bulimia, anorexia, and obesity have been associated with or traced to allergies.

Suprisingly enough, addictions have been linked with allergies. Stephen Levine, Ph.D., has made this observation: "Allergy or allergic-like sensitivities nearly always accompany addiction. Allergy may occur without addiction but, generally, addiction is always accompanied by allergy. Alcoholics, smokers, and coffee drinkers are allergic to the very substances they crave. 'Allergy-Addiction syndrome' has been used to describe this phenomenon...Addiction-prone individuals, because of their basic physiological makeup, are more likely to overuse cigarettes, coffee, milk, wheat, or common foods to satisfy their constant need for stimulation. Any subtle signal of withdrawl symptoms triggers the individual to eat the necessary food or have a cigarette. The increasing addictive nature of these substances continues in a vicious cycle. When an individual forces himself to give up one substance, alcohol for example, he may in compensation, increase his consumption of coffee, cigarettes, and addictive foods. In this manner, the stimulated state is maintained and withdrawl symptoms avoided. Only when regular consumptom of all addictants is stopped can a symptom-free state be established. The best testing procedure involves a single food rotation diet where a particular food is avoided until a full four-day period has elapsed. After four days of avoiding repetitive use of an addictant the body will regain its normal ability to discriminate an allergen from an addictant. The addicted state is now over. The body has regained a form of intelligence and will react acutely to harmful substances. When you experience an acute reaction to a previously favorite food or drug, it is convincing evidence of prior addiction."

Undigested proteins act as irritants in the body. The T-cells treat them as foreign invaders, thus inviting an "allergic attack." An efficient digestive capability is necessary to prevent accumulations of these substances in the bloodstream. Mucous membranes line many areas of the body, the nose, throat most organs and glands, and the gastrointestinal tract. Healthy mucous membranes will not allow the undigested proteins to enter the bloodstream. Herbs have the ability to protect these mucous membranes.   *Slows the heart   raises the blood pressure*

Ephedra, white willow bark, lobelia, goldenseal root, bee pollen, capsicum, chaparral. Bee Pollen should always be started in small amounts at first. Burdock, comfrey, echinacea, fenugreek, ma heung (natural antihistamine *decongestant*), scullcap, hops, gotu kola.   *chinese ephedra*

An herbal lung combination to build up the lungs and lower bowel combination will help in allergies.

In *The Ultimate Healing System,* by Donald LePore, N.D., he suggests about allergies that, "part of the solution to the problem first is to find out why the adrenal cortex is malfunctioning. The malfunctioning can occur due to: A) A lack of Pantothenic Acid in the system causing a citrus allergy; B) A lack of Potassium causing an allergy to milk, cheese, green and all sodium foods. C) A lack of sodium which can create allergies to everything. With these deficiencies and allergies present, sugars are not absorbed properly by the body."

The adrenal cortex can be normalized by:

A) Pantothenic Acid (Vitmain B5), which can be found in abundance in "Royal Jelly". It is also found in barberry, parsley, kelp, hops, gotu kola, papaya, peppermint, ginseng, slippery elm and spirulina. _bad for people with Lupus_

B) Potassium, which is found naturally in alfalfa and bee pollen. Also found in kelp, valerian, stevia, scullcap, red clover, parsley and garlic. _herbal (green) sweetener_

C) Sodium, which is found in alfalfa and spirulina. Also found in chickweed, buchu, burdock, gotu kola, safflower, rosehips sarsaparilla, peppermint, papaya, parsley, licorice and dandelion. _diuretic laxative, blood pressure raiser_

DIGESTION AND HYPOGLYCEMIA

Most digestion and assimilation takes place in the twenty five feet of small intestine, which is located between the stomach and the large bowel, or colon.

The small intestine is lined with a mucus membrane, designed with orifices, or small openings which permit passage of digested foods to penetrate through the wall.

If elimination has been sluggish, and the diet is void of roughage, the gentle abrasion of stimulation of the membrane is insufficient to keep it cleaned and functional. The undue pressure forces the small openings to become enlarged, permitting incomplete digested food to migrate into the bloodstream. If protein is allowed to remain too long in the intestine, bacteria will have an opportunity to act upon it. Tyrosin will be converted to phenol, tryptophan to indole and skatole. Phenol is both a local corrosive and a systemic poison which can kill cells.

Protein deficiency or incomplete protein digestion are related to most degenerative conditions. This is the reason that a high protein diet is not beneficial for any disease, especially hypoglycemia.

Uric acid is the waste product of protein metabolism. It contains purine (similar to caffeine) which is a known stimulant. The body can eliminate about 8 grams of uric acid daily. Any build-up of excess uric acid accumulates in the blood and tissues of the body causing toxemia, kidney problems, arthritis, gout, along with many other diseases.

31

MEAT

Meat is hard to digest and it takes about 6 hours. It puts a burden on the organs of the body. It is also hard to assimilate and eliminate. It contains no fiber to keep it moving through the intestines. It takes longer than any other food to go through the intestines. It begins to ferment and putrify producing acids and gases. Meat has been directly connected to colon problems, such as colon cancer, colitis and diverticulosis. Meat is high in phosphorus and leaches calcium from the bones. It creates an nutritional imbalance in the body.

Most meat today is tainted, chemicalized with antibiotics and hormones, and adulterated from sick and overmedicated animals. Steer which has been penned up for months at a time suffer from cancer or tuberculosis. Antibiotics and steroid hormones in the feed, is added to prevent infections and increase weight quickly.

A high protein diet can control the symptoms of hypoglycemia but is it worth it? It can lead to many serious biochemical and metabolic disorders. It can contribute to diseases such as arthritis, osteoporosis, periodontal disease, heart disease, cancer and many other diseases. It can cause toxic blood, hormone imbalance, constipation, exhaustion, headaches, lack of energy, mental and physical sluggishness.

CHIROPRACTIC OR REFLEXOLOGY TREATMENTS

Many who have suffered from hypoglycemia have found that some type of massage therapy is excellent to help control it along with diet, herbs, vitamins and minerals. Along with stress management and exercise.

With hypoglycemia the body usually has chronic muscle tension, either in the jaws, neck, shoulders, head and etc. Some feel that the most common cause of low blood sugar is the tensed muscles. Spasm of a muscle is continually working and burning fuel. Since sugar is the fuel and stored in the muscle cells, it is possible that tensed muscles could create problems in hypoglycemia.

Spasms of the muscles can be broken with body therapy and create relaxation. Deep massage in tension spots will relax muscles and help elevate stress. This will also relax the pancreas, and help it do its job. An adrenal weakness is often experienced as a deep ache in the small of the back. Aching joints are one of the first signs of adrenal exhaustion.

Those with hypoglycemia seem to always be in a tense state. They are usually the most dynamic, motivated people around us. They usually demand perfection in everything. These type of people usually push themselves to excel and work too hard at a fast pace and eat the wrong kinds of food and suffer a "burn out" and total lowering of nerve energy. It becomes a constant cycle, becoming angry, or fall into a deep despair which will drain vital nerve energy even more.

EXERCISE

Exercise is very important to lower blood cholesterol, and normalize blood sugar. Walking and deep breathing are also very beneficial. Regualr exercise moves blood sugar into the body's cells, providing energy, without requiring insulin.

Exercise "burns off" excess adrenalin and thereby reduces the symptoms of stress. It improves circulation, increases oxygen reserves, strengthens the heart, lungs and glandular system.

Exercise also helps to keep appetite under control.

VITAMINS FOR HYPOGLYCEMIA

Vitamin A - Assists in maintaining normal glandular function. Energy transfer in the body depends upon vitamin A. Use with vitamin D and E to help in proper assimilation. Protects the mucous membranes. Helps in assimilation of minerals.

Vitamin B-Complex - A natural high potency vitamin B complex is excellent. They are necessary to help control hypoglycemia's highs and lows. They build the adrenals, and calm the nerves.

Vitamin B1 (Thiamine) - Assists in metabolizing carbohydrates, improves appetite, digestion, assimilation and elimination. Protects the nervous system and improves nerve function.

Vitamin B2 (Riboflavin) - Works with niacin and thiamine. Protects the nerves and immune system. Promotes a healthy digestive tract.

Vitamin B3 (Niacinamide) - Essential for production of male and female sex hormones. Helps to regulate blood sugar levels in hypoglycemia. Used to treat schizophrenic and austistic children. Promotes appetite, digestion, assimilation and elimination.

Vitamin B5 (Panthothenic Acid) - Deficiency of this vitmain could cause low blood sugar as well as a rapid drop in sugar levels. This B vitamin is directly involved in the production of natural cortisone. Protects against stress, calms the nerves. Essential for health of adrenals glands and hormone production.

Vitamin B6 (Pyridoxine Hydrochloride) - Builds the adrenals and protects the pancreas. Protects against stress. Helps in prevention of motion sickness, nausea and morning sickness in pregnancy. Necessary for glucose tolerance. It is essential for metabolism of proteins, production of antibodies, hormone adrenalin to maintain mineral balance. It helps in the conversion of oxalic acid into a harmless form.

Vitamin B9 (Folic Acid) - Necessary for liver enzyme to function effectively. Essential for the formation of new red blood cells, production of antibodies and the maintenance of the reproductive glands. Essential for the absorption of iron and calcium with B12 and vitamin C to break down protein.

Vitamin B12 (Cobalamin) - Protects the liver which is often toxic and overstressed in hypoglycemia. Helps eliminate cholesterol, protects the nervous system from deterioration. Essential in the metabolism of carbohydrate, fat and protein, Improves brain function.

Vitamin B13 (Orotic Acid) - Necessary for a healthy nervous system and proper brain function.

Vitamin B15 (Pangamic Acid) - Supplies oxygen to living cells. Builds the immune system. Stimulates the glandular and nervous system. Protects the body against cancer.

Vitamin B17 (Laetrile) - Believed to have cancer controlling and preventive properties that literally poison the malignant cell while nourishing all other cells. *If it nourishes the other cells then why will it kill you if you eat too much?*

34

PABA (Para-aminobenzoic Acid) - Aids in produciton of pantothenic acid, which builds the adrenals. Enhances intestinal flora and health of intestines.

Choline - Strengthens blood capillaries, aids in eliminating cholesterol from the blood. Aids in digestion of fatty foods. Necessary for storage of minerals, especially calcium and vitamin A.

Inositol - Reduces blood cholesterol, and cleans excessive fat from the blood. Stimulates digestion. Necessary to stimulate normal growth and survival of cells in the bone marrow and eye membranes. Protects against eye problems.

Lecithin - Helps to protect the veins, nervous system and brain. Helps regulate metabolism and break down fat and cholesterol and prevent it from adhering to the artery walls.

Vitamin C - Promotes normal adrenal function and glandular activity. Concentration is in the adrenal glands. Helps to prevent low blood sugar attacks. It is known that personality changes occurs at a state of vitamin C depletion well before obvious clinical scurvy is evident. Plays an important role in sugar metabolism.

Vitamin D - Essential for health of glandular and nervous system. Regulated mineral and vitamin metabolism, especially calcium, Vitamin A and phosphorus. Protects the immune system.

Vitamin E - Essential for health of adrenal and pituitary glands. Helps strengthen and tone muscles, protects the lungs, prevents sterility, and protects against radiation. It protects the B vitamins from rapid oxidation. Reduces cholesterol.

Vitamin F (Unsaturated Fatty Acids) - Essential for proper function of the adrenal and thyroid glands. Protects the veins, increases circulation, reduces cholesterol and assists in retaining fat soluble vitamins in the system. Lubricates the cells for healthy tone and elasticity.

Vitamin H (Biotin) - Essential for metabolism of carbohydrates, fat and

35

protein. Necessary for utilization of B complex vitamins. Necessary for all glandular secretions, fatty acid production, male sex hormones and the nerves.

Vitamin K - Necessary for conversion of carbohydrates into glucose. Helps blood to clot. Important for normal function of the heart and liver. *Do not take this if the Dr. has you on blood thinners or if you clot too easily*

Vitamin P (Bioflavonoids) - Increases effectiveness of vitamin C, prevents and heals bleeding gums. Builds the immune system. Helps in maintaining healthy capillaries.

MINERALS FOR HYPOGLYCEMIA

Calcium - Improves acid-alkaline balance. To function effeciently calcium must be in combination with magnesium, phosphorus, vitamin A, D, and C as well as zinc and inositol for proper absorption. It must also have an acid environment, otherwise it can collect in the joints and tissues. *Boron helps too*

Chlorine - Helps to regulate hormone distribution throughout the body. It expells waste, purifies and disinfects, fights germs and bacteria and assists liver in filtering toxins.

Chromium - Essential for correct sugar metabolism. Plays a vital role in the breakdown of sucrose to dextrose and fructose.

Iodine - Essential for regulating the thyroid gland to manufacture the hormone thyroxin to control metabolism in the body. Regulates cholesterol levels. Protects against toxins in the brain. Found naturally in kelp, dulse, black walnut and spirulina.

Magnesium - Helps prevent adrenal instability. Keeps calcium from depositing in arteries, joints and cells. It is necessary to pump the calcium out of the cells. Magnesium decreases the need for calcium. Helps in the conversion of blood sugar to energy. Helps the nervous system, prevents depression. Found in nuts, whole grains, greens, berries, and yellow corn.

Manganese - Assists in pancreatic development, and in maintenance of the central nervous system. Activates enzymes to convert lactate and alanine into glucose.

Potassium - Helps regulate blood sugar. Helps the body to handle stress. Usually lacking in those with hypoglycemia. Potassium is called the healing mineral. All glands can heal quicker when potssium is added. It is found in kelp, dulse, and irish moss.

Selenium - works with vitamin E to help the body utilize oxygen. Helps protect against toxic build-up in the body.

Silicon - Helps strengthen the body, especially the bones. A cleansing mineral.

Zinc - It is involved with the systems ability to utilize insulin. It is often lacking in hypoglycemics. Without zinc the "insulin" burns too fast and depletes the blood sugar.

AMINO ACIDS

Alanine - Strengthens cellular walls and helps the liver to detoxify toxins.

Carnitine - Contributes to glucose function. It has been suggested that it may be an early symptom of hypoglycemia if there is a deficiency of carnitine. It enables the muscles to utilize fatty acids for energy.

Glutamic Acid - Helps curb cravings for refined sugar. It is considered a brain food.

Phynylalanine and Tyrosine - Responsible for adrenalin, which is produced by the adrenal glands.

HERBS FOR HYPOGLYCEMIA

Herbs for the glandular system help to regulate and balance body function. Healthy glands are vital to help all systems to operate efficiently, manufacture vital substances, such as hormones, to store certain elements and to detoxify the body's blood and lymph fluids. The herbs help keep the bloodstream clean, cells in healthy condition and prevent germs and toxins from multiplying.

The systems in the body that need special attention, to have a healthy glandular system are: Glandular, ciruclatory, digestive, and nervous.

Glandular System - Alfalfa, black walnut, burdock, chickweed, chaparral, dandelion, echinacea, ephedra, golden seal, kelp, lobelia, licorice, oregon grape, peach bark, red clover, sarsaparilla, yarrow, yellow dock, yucca, watercress, wild yam.

means raises blood pressure

Circulatory System - Bugleweed, butchers broom, capsicum, cloves, ephedra, garlic, gentian, ginger, gotu kola, hawthorn, mistletoe, passion flower, rosemary, siberian ginseng, vervain, watercress, yarrow.

means dangerous if given in any but tiny amounts

Digestive System - Alfalfa, barberry, comfrey, dandelion, gentian, ginger, golden seal, irish moss, kelp, marshmallow, myrrh, slippery elm, wormwood.

Nervous System - Black cohosh, chamomile, damiana, gotu kola, hops, ho-sho-wu, lady's slipper, lobelia, misteltoe, passion flower, scullcap, St. Johnswort, siberian ginseng, valerian root, vervain, wild lettuce, wood betony.

HERBAL BENEFITS FOR THE GLANDS

Alfalfa: Nourishing and cleansing for all the glands but especially beneficial for the pituitary gland. Provides vegetable protein which is essential for the health of the glands.

Black Cohosh: A female hormone herb, it has many uses, relieves spasms, cramps, balances hormones. Stimulates estrogen production.

Blessed Thistle: Balances hormones. Provides nutrition for the female reproductive system.

Buchu: Rich in potassium (the healing mineral), heals swollen prostate gland. *Found in diuretics*

Cedar Berries: Heals and nourishes the pancreas. Acts as a diuretic and like golden seal, it promotes natural insulin function. Natural antibiotic.

Chamomile: Soothes the nerves and aids digestion.

Damiana: Tonic for the reproductive organs, nerves and kidneys. Historically used to strengthen the male sexual organs. Contains properties to stimulate the male hormone testosterone.

Dandelion: Cleans the liver and helps to balance blood sugar.

Dong Quai: Nourishes the female glands. It is very nourishing to the brain and strengthens the central nervous system.

Dulse: Rich in iodine, which nourishes the thyroid and other glands.

Ginseng: Helps the body maintain adrenal levels. Nourishing to the whole body. Increases vitality and energy. Regenerates and rebuilds the male sex glands.

Gentian: Tonic to strengthen a weakened digestive tract, including the liver.

Golden Seal: Helps to regulate blood sugar levels. Many have gotten off insulin by slowly adding golden seal. It is considered the "cure-all" herb. *But 1) it raises b.p. & 2) it should only be taken for 10 days in a row.*

Ho-Sho-Wu: Tonic for the endocrine glands. Improves stamina and resistance to disease.

Kelp: Contains iodine which is essential to the restoration of the pituitary, adrenal, pineal, thyroid and parathyroid glands. Burns fat, cleans the veins, nourishes the whole body. Regulates the adrenal and pituitary glands.

Licorice: Acts in the body like the cortin hormone and protects the body by helping to cope with stress. It allows the blood sugar level to remain normal and provide a feeling of well-being. An important herb for the adrenal glands. Provides nutrients to promote the secretion of adrenalin. *It leads to water retention it can lead to high blood pressure*

Lobelia: It will remove obstructions wherever they are located in the body. It is one of the greatest herbs in the herbal kingdom. It relaxes the body. It helps to clean the glands. *It slows down the heart. Slow it down too much, you're dead*

Mullein: Beneficial to clean and nourish the glands. Along with lobelia, a great gland booster. Helps to balance hormone secretions.

Parsley: Supplies potassium, sodium and magnesium, essential for glandular health. Activates enzymes in the body. Helps in the process of carbohydrate metabolism, protein synthesis and energy transfer. It contains traces of copper, chromium, cobalt and zinc which nourishes the adrenal glands. *diuretic. Good for the Liver*

Red Raspberry: Regulates acid/alkaline balance in the body and in blood sugar imbalances. Helps to maintain energy levels.

Saffron: Allows the body to regulate the lactic acid and to utilize oils. It has a beneficial effect on the duodenum, gall bladder and the liver.

Sarsaparilla: Balances hormones. Cleans the blood. Strengthens the immune system.

Saw Palmetto: Helps control and normalize the function of the pancreas, the adrenals as well as all vital organs and glands. Rich in iron, enzymes, amino acids, and carbohydrates. *good for the prostate gland*

Suma: An herb beneficial to both men and women to restore sexual function. Also helps in poor circulation, heart disease and arthritis. Contains germanium, a trace mineral which enhances the immune system.

Uva Ursi: Helps to regulate glucose transfer to the nerve fiber to feed the brain. *diuretic*

HELPFUL HINTS

Avoid the following alkaloids, they are a toxic alkaloid group that damage the pancreas. These are products that can interfere with the glandular function. They can become addictive and create a craving.

NICOTINE (tobacco)
CAFFEINE (coffee, soft drinks)
THEOBROMINE (chocolate, cocoa)
THEOPHYLLINE (tea)
PURINES (found in certain animal products, coffee, mate tea, teas, chocolate)

Chocolate and caffeine together seem to produce an addiction in the body. Caffeine and nicotine stimulates insulin production. Caffeine injures the islets of langerhans in the pancreas where insulin is produced.

Carbonated drinks interfere with digestion. Stomach problems are frequent with hypoglycemia.

Avoid heavy fat diets. Diets low in fats cause a lowering of the blood sugar in hypoglycemia, and a reduction of sugar in the urine.

Avoid an excess of dairy products. High in lactose (mild sugar), constipating, and builds excess mucous in the body, which breeds germs and viruses.

Avoid disguised sweetners. Read labels. The following are forms of sugars. Dextrose, Dextrin, Maltose (cereal sugar), Lactose (milk sugar), Sucrose (table sugar), Fructose (fruit sugar), Modified food starch, Cornstarch, Corn syrup, Corn sweetener, Natural sweetener, Honey (use in small amounts), Molasses (use in small amounts). The following are alcohols, and the body reacts to as them as with refined carbohydrates: Sorbitol, mannitol, hexitol, glycol.

Avoid too much table salt. It creates adrenal exhaustion. It causes a loss of potassium which leads to a drop in blood sugar. Potassium is necessary to restore sugar metabolism abnormalities.

SUGGESTED GUIDLINES

1. Discontinue eating food that cause the problems in the first place.

White flour and white sugar products. Refined, and processed foods. Fast foods cooked in rancid oils. Heavy meat diets, ice cream, pastries, cookies, candy, processed cereals, soft drinks, caffeine products.

2. Eat less at each meal. Food will digest better. Realize that food should be seen as nutritional and not entertainment. *dorn*

3. Learn stress reduction. Learn to be happy. Develop a regular exercise program. Enjoy fresh air out of doors. Get more sunlight.

4. Emphasize more whole grains (millet, buckwheat, rye, wheat, barley), raw seeds, raw nuts, beans, vegetables and fruit. Use sprouts a lot, they will heal and provide nutrients to combat hypoglycemia. Grains digest very slowly and release sugar into the blood stream gradually for as long as 6 to 8 hours after the meal. It helps to keep blood sugar level constant for a long period of time.

Grains, seeds and nuts are also rich in the minerals magnesium, zinc and manganese, all the vital nutrients for prevention and treatment of hypoglycemia.

The United States Department of Agriculture has verified that the protein in buckwheat is complete and superior to meat.

SEVEN-DAY SUGGESTED MENU

Nutritional supplements, such as vitamins, minerals and herbs are best taken with meals. If digestion is a problem, digestive enzymes and hydrochloric acid can be added. Herbal teas are very beneficial to purify the bloodstream. Use often: Red clover, alfalfa, pau d'arco, red raspberry and licorice.

The ideal diet for hypoglycemia is one designed to promote good health as well as prevent the disease. It would consist of natural complex carbohydrates, such as grains, seeds, nuts, vegetables, fruits and some dairy products and small amounts of meat, fish and poultry. A diet low in protein, low in fat and high in natural carbohydrates is ideal. Eat a variety of nourishing foods. Sprouts should be high on the list.

MENU

Before breakfast a glass of pure water with ½ fresh lemon juice, or water with 2 tablespoons of liquid chlorophyll and 2 Tab. aloe vera juice, or a green drink. Protein powder can also be added.

GREEN DRINK

4 oz. of pineapple juice or fresh apple juice
4 oz. pure water
2 oz. aloe vera juice
2 large comfrey leaves
½ cup sprouts
¼ cup parsley.

Blend well and drink before breakfast.

#1 Breakfast
1 ripe peach
*Oatmeal cereal

#1 Lunch
*Baked potato with chili stuffing
Large Green salad (Leaf lettuce with 6 raw vegetables)

#1 Supper
*Almond and bean salad
Raw vegetable plate
1 slice rye bread

#2 Breakfast
1 small green apple (30 minutes before breakfast)
*Seed cereal

#2 Lunch
*Chicken salad

#2 Supper
*Brown rice special

#3 Breakfast
1 pear
*Cornmeal cereal

#3 Lunch
Pocket bread sandwith (whole wheat)
Use you imagination: avaocado, onions, tomatoes, green peppers, little cheese, sprouts, grated carrots, mayonaise.

#3 Supper
*Enchilladas
Green salad

#4 Breakfast
2 apricots (or other fruit)
*Seed cereal

#4 Lunch
*Brown rice and almond dish
1 slice whole wheat bread

#4 Supper
*Baked chicken breast
Raw vegetables (carrots, zucchini, celery)
Steamed broccoli

#5 Breakfast
1 Bran muffin
2 soft boiled fertile eggs

#5 Lunch
*Pinto bean soup
Green salad (with sprouts)

#5 Supper
*Quinoa supper
Steamed vegetables (greenbeans, carrots and summer squash)

#6 Breakfast
½ cup - raspberries
*Brown rice (cooked in thermos)

#6 Lunch
Baked potato (with butter & chives)
*Mixed vegetable salad
1 slice rye bread

#6 Supper
*Kasha supreme
Corn bread

#7 Breakfast
1 tangerine
*Whole wheat and buckwheat pancakes
(blender method)
¼ tea. pure maple syrup

#7 Lunch
*Rice and corn salad
1 slice rye bread

#7 Supper
*Burrito Dinner

RECIPES

OATMEAL CEREAL
Soak overnight

½ cup whole oats or baby oats
1 Tab. sesame seeds
6 almonds
1 tea. chia seeds
1 tea. flax seeds

Try to eat it unsweetened. A few drops of pure maple syrup can be added.

SEED CEREAL
Rich in protein, calcium and packed with lasting energy. Combine the following and keep in a jar in refrigerator.

1 cup sesame seeds
1 cup chia seeds
1 cup sunflower seeds
1 cup flax seeds
1 cup pumpkin seeds

Take two to four tablespoons and soak in pure water overnight. Next morning, blend in blender and add to grape nuts or any unsweetened cereal, or eat alone.

CORNMEAL CEREAL
Cornmeal is a laxative starch and is high in magnesium that is useful in constipation. It will not produce catarrh. Yellow corn meal is best.

¼ cup cornmeal
1 cup pure water

Boil water and gradually add to boiling water. Cover and cook for about 30 minutes. You can also cook overnight in a thermos.

BROWN RICE

½ cup basmiti brown rice (Smells like pop corn when cooking)
1 cup boiling water

Pour boiling water over rice in wide mouth thermos. Cook overnight.

WHOLE WHEAT AND BUCKWHEAT PANCAKES

½ cup whole wheat berries
¼ cup buckwheat (hulled)
1 cup milk (almond milk or powdered milk)

Blend at high speed for four minutes. Add dash salt, 2 tea. baking powder, 2 eggs and ¼ cup oil. Blend all together and cook like pancakes.

LUNCH

BAKED POTATO WITH CHILI STUFFING

1 Baked potato per person
Chili Sauce
1½ tea. oil (light olive oil)
2 clove garlic
¼ pound of ground turkey (optional)
1 cup cooket pinto beans
1 Tab. chili powder
Cayenne and kelp to taste
½ cup tomato sauce
Grated cheese

Heat oil and saute onion garlic and turkey. Stir until meat is brown. Add beans, chili powder, cayenne and kelp.

Half baked potatoes lengthwise. Scoop out half of flesh. Fill each shell with meat mixture. Top each with 2 tablespoons tomato sauce, and grated cheese. Place filled shells in a baking dish and bake in oven at 350 degrees for 30 minutes.

CHICKEN SALAD

1 cup fresh bean sprouts
1 cup alfalfa sprouts
1 cup shredded cabbage
1 Tab. soy sauce
2 tea. wine vinegar
2 tea. light olive oil
½ cup grated carrots
¼ cup green onions
8 ounces cooked chicken breast, cubed

Combine all ingredients except chicken and toss thoroughly. Add chicken and toss lightly. Makes 2 large servings.

BROWN RICE AND ALMOND DISH

2 Tab. light olive oil
1¾ cups vegetable broth
1 clove garlic
1 tea. marjoran, crushed
1 cup zucchini squash
1 cup carrots, grated
1 Tab. arrowroot powder
1 cup cherry tomatoes
½ cup green onions, chopped
½ cup almonds, ground
2 cups cooked brown basamiti rice

Saute in heated stainless steel wok, olive oil and garlic. Add broth, simmer for ten minutes. Add marjorim, squash, carrots and arrowroot powder blended with 2 tablespoons water. Stir and cook until sauce thickens. Add tomatoes, onions, and almonds and cook for one minute. Serve over hot rice. Serves about 4.

PINTO BEAN MEAL

1 cup cooked buckwheat
1 med. onion
1 16 oz. can tomato puree
1 16 oz. can pure water
¼ cup green chilis
2 clove garlic
1 tea. cumin
3 cups cooked pinto beans
Dash of chili powder

Saute buckwheat, onion and garlic in medium saucepan. Add tomato puree and water. Season with cumin and a dash of chili powder. Simmer for 30 minutes. Add pinto beans.

MIXED VEGETABLE SALAD

1 medium bermuda onion, peeled and cut in paper-thin slices
2 medium ripe tomatoes, sliced in chunks
Bunch of red radishes. Washed and cut in half
1 head butter lettuce
1 Tab. fresh lemon juice
½ tea. cayenne pepper
1 Tab. light olive oil

Toss all together and serve.

RICE AND CORN SALAD

2 cups cooked brown rice
2 cups fresh corn kernels
1 cup cherry tomatoes, sliced in half
½ cup chopped green pepper
½ cup chopped green onions
½ cup black olives, sliced
½ cup chopped fresh parsley basil and dill

DRESSING:
2 Tab. wine vinegar
2 Tab. water
2 Tab. soy sauce, natural
½ tea. Dijon mustard
Dash cayenne pepper

Combine salad ingredients. Combine dressing ingredients in a small jar. Pour over salad. Mix well. Serves 6 to 8. If there is any left over it is even better it chills in refrigerator for several hours. Good for supper.

SUPPER

ALMOND AND BEAN SALAD

4 cups fresh green beans, washed, stem and cut in thin pieces
1 cup almonds, sliced thin
1 medium onion, chopped
2½ Tab. light olive oil
2 Tab. butter
1 Tab. Tamari sauce
1 Tab. white wine vinegar
1 Cup alfalfa and fenugreek sprouts
For garnish:
Tomato wedges
Fresh parsley, chopped
Fresh dill and basil

Saute greens beans in frying pan with oil and onions. Cook for about 15 minutes. Add tamari and stir for 1 minute. Remove from fire add almonds and vinegar. Serve in salad bowl with alfalfa sprouts, tomatoes and fresh parsley, dill and basil.

BROWN RICE SPECIAL

2 Tab. butter
2 Tab. light olive oil
2 Clove garlic, minced
1 Cup onion, chopped
1 Cup green pepper, chopped
2 Cups cooked brown basmati rice.
½ Cup raw almonds, ground
2 Tab. worcestershire sauce
3 Tab. toasted sesame seeds

Saute together, butter, oil, garlic, onion and green pepper. Cook slightly, they should be crunchy. Add rice until heated. Add almonds, worchestershire sauce and sesame seeds, cook for a few minutes. Ready to serve. Serves about 4 people.

ENCHILLADAS

3 cups cooked pinto beans
½ cup chopped onion
2 clove garlic
1 small can green chilies
½ can tomato puree
¼ can enchillada sauce
2 Tab. vegetable seasoning in ½ cup water
½ tea. cumin
½ tea. chili powder
Cheese, grated
Sour cream, or mock sour cream

Mash cooked pinto beans. Saute onions, garlic and green chilies. Add cumin, chili powder. Add vegetable seasoning, water and tomato puree and enchilladas sauce. It should be very thick. Roll this mixture in corn tortillas. Add cheese and a little sour cream before rolling up.

SAUCE

¾ can of enchillada sauce (left over from above)
½ can tomato puree (from above)
½ cup onion, minced
½ cup water with vegetable seasoning to taste
1 tea. chili powder
Pinch of garlic powder and onion powder

Simmer on low for 30 minutes. Pour over enchilladas and bake for about 30 minutes at 350 degrees.

BAKED CHICKEN BREAST

Boneless, skinless chicken breast
(for how ever many are eating)
Dip cold chicken in warm olive oil and butter.
Cover with seasoned bread crumbs.
Bake in oven for about 45 minutes.

QUINOA SUPPER

(KEEN-wa) A new powerful grain, with a gourmet flavor. Easy to digest. Good for allergy-prone individuals.

1 cup Quinoa
2 cups pure water
½ cup grated carrots
½ cup broccoli, chopped fine
1 cup fresh corn
½ cup almonds, ground
1 Tab. butter
2 Tab. light olive oil
1 large onion
2 clove garlic

Toast quinoa in a pan with a teaspoonful of olive oil for a few minutes until it turns darker. Add to boiling water and cook for about 30 minutes.
Saute in butter and olive oil, onion and garlic.
Add the carrots, broccoli, corn and almonds to quinoa when done and serve.

KASHA SUPREME

1 large onion, chopped
2 clove garlic
2 Tab. olive oil
2 Tab. butter
1 egg, slightly beaten
1 cup kasha (roasted buckwheat kernels)
2 cups water
2 tea. vegetable seasoning
1 cup cottage cheese
1 cup fresh or frozen corn
1 cup cheddar cheese, grated
¼ cup diced red pepper
1 cup cherry tomatoes, cut in half

Saute onion and garlic in olive oil and butter for about 10 minutes. Stir egg into kasha in small bowl, add to onion. stirring constantly until each grain separates. Stir in water and vegetable seasoning, bring to boil, and lower heat, cover and cook for about 20 minutes.

Mix cottage cheese, corn red pepper and cheddar cheese. Put in oven in a glass dish and cook until cheese melts. Garnish with tomatoes. Ready to eat.

BURRITO DINNER

1 large onion, chopped
1 large carrot, grated
1 stalk celery, chopped
1 green pepper, chopped
½ cup green onions, chopped
1 Tab. light olive oil or sunflower seed oil
2 clove garlic, pressed
1½ cups corn (fresh or frozen)
2 cups cooked pinto beans
1 Tab. chili powder
1 tea. oregano
¼ tea. cayenne powder
¼ cup water

ALSO: Chopped tomatoes, shredded leaf lettuce, green onions, sprouts and your favorite salsa to put on burritos.

Where is the beef?

Saute first five ingredients in oil for 10 minutes. Add remaining ingredients and mix carefully. Bring to boil, cover, reduce heat and cook over medium-low heat for 20 minutes. Check and stir occasionally. Serves 4 to 6. Fill tortilla. You can also serve this over brown rice.

FURTHER READING

Airola, Paavo, Ph.D., *Hypoglycemia. A Better Approach.*

Barmakian, Richard, N.D., *Hypoglycemia Your Bondage or Freedom.*

Barnes, Broda O., M.D., Ph.D., and Barnes, Charlotte W. A.M., *Hope For Hypoglycemia.*

Tenney, Louise, M.H., *Today's Herbal Health, Today's Healthy Eating, Modern Day Plagues, Health Handbook* and *Today's Herbs, newsletter.*